Positive Affirmations
Coloring Book

Aryla Publishing 2021

978-1-912675-97-5

www.arylapublishing.com

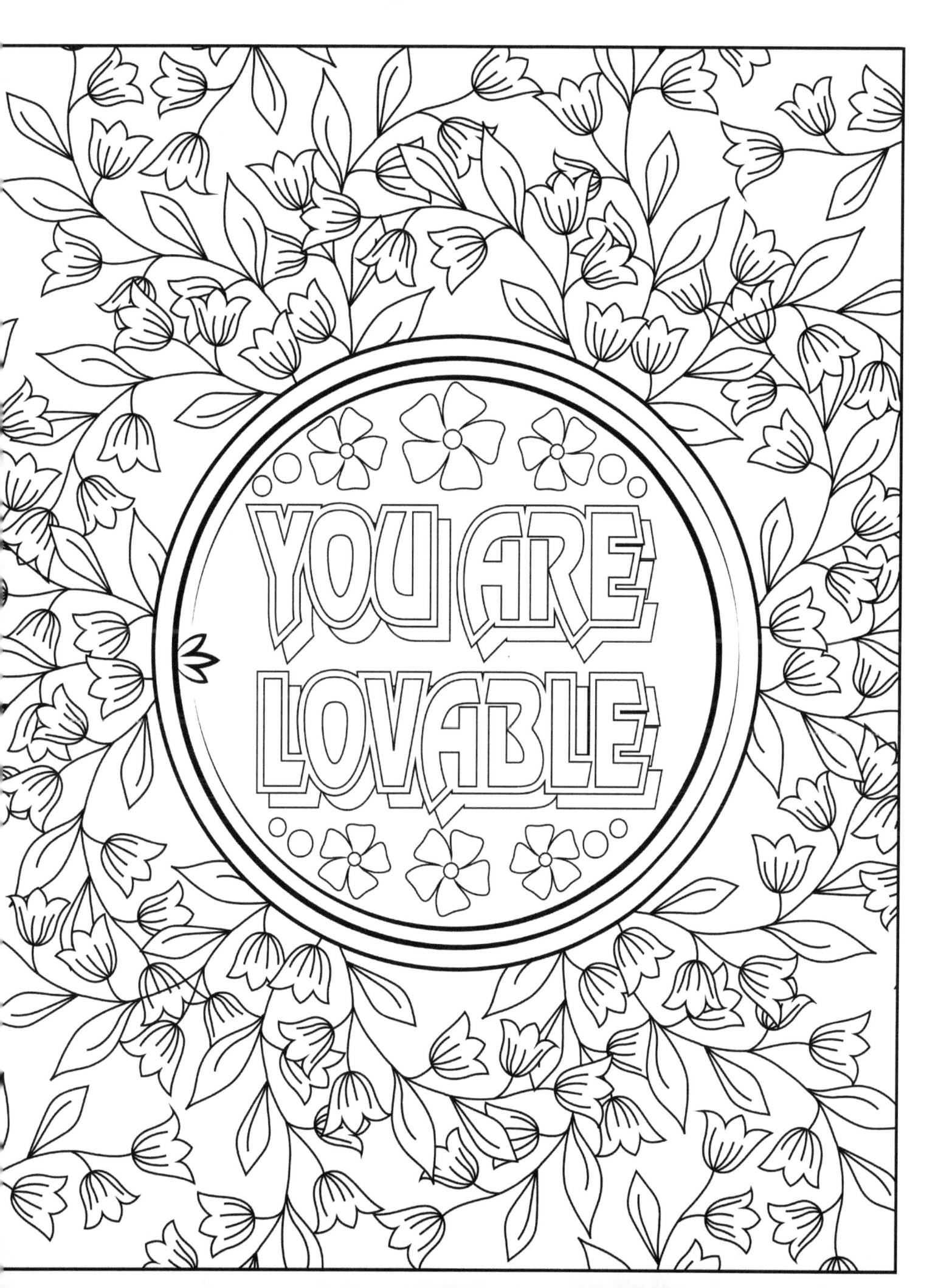

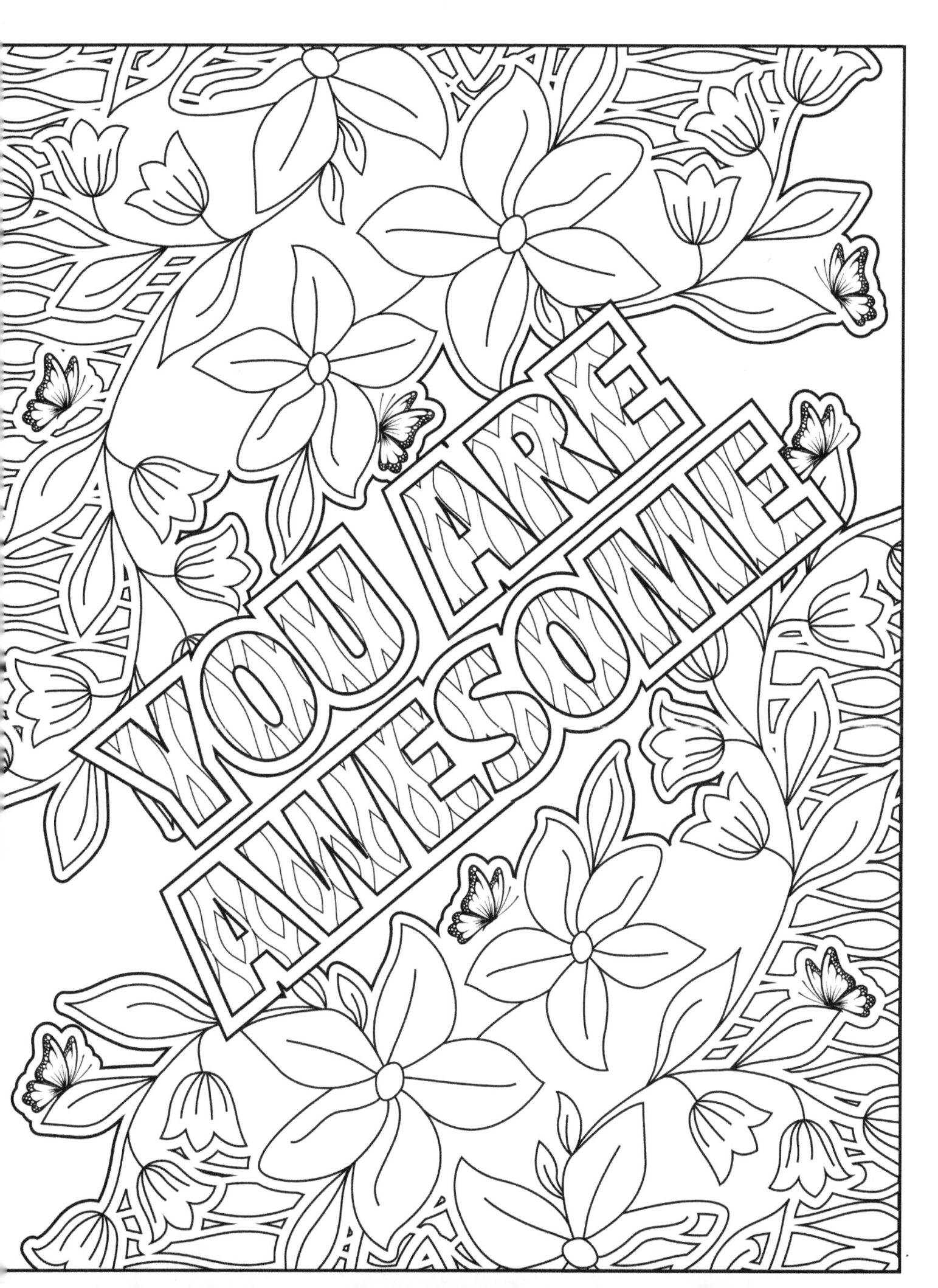

YOU ARE WORTHY

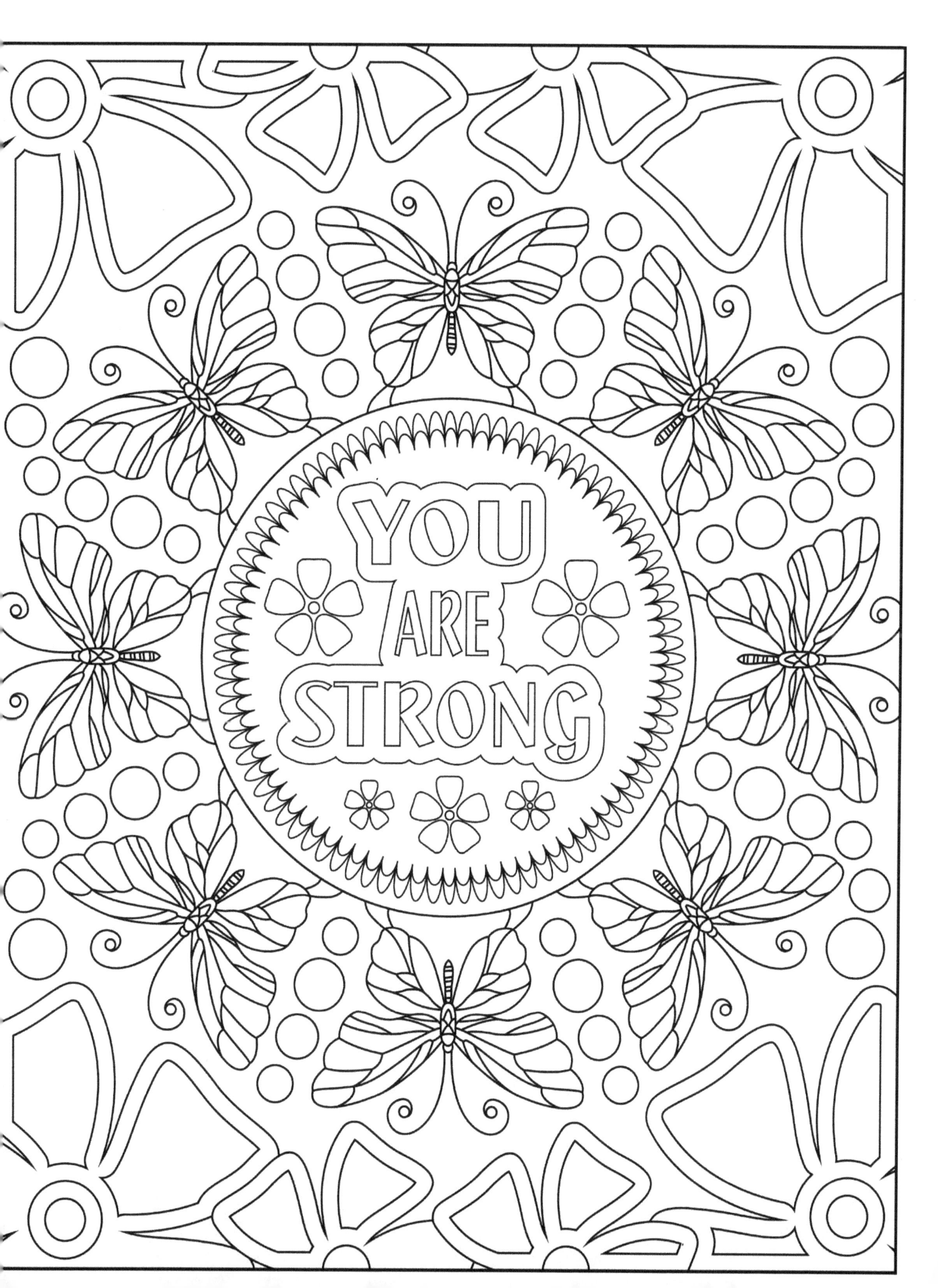

YOU
ARE
STRONG

TRUST YOUR WISE VOICE WITHIN

BE COURAGEOUS WITH YOUR GENTLE HEART

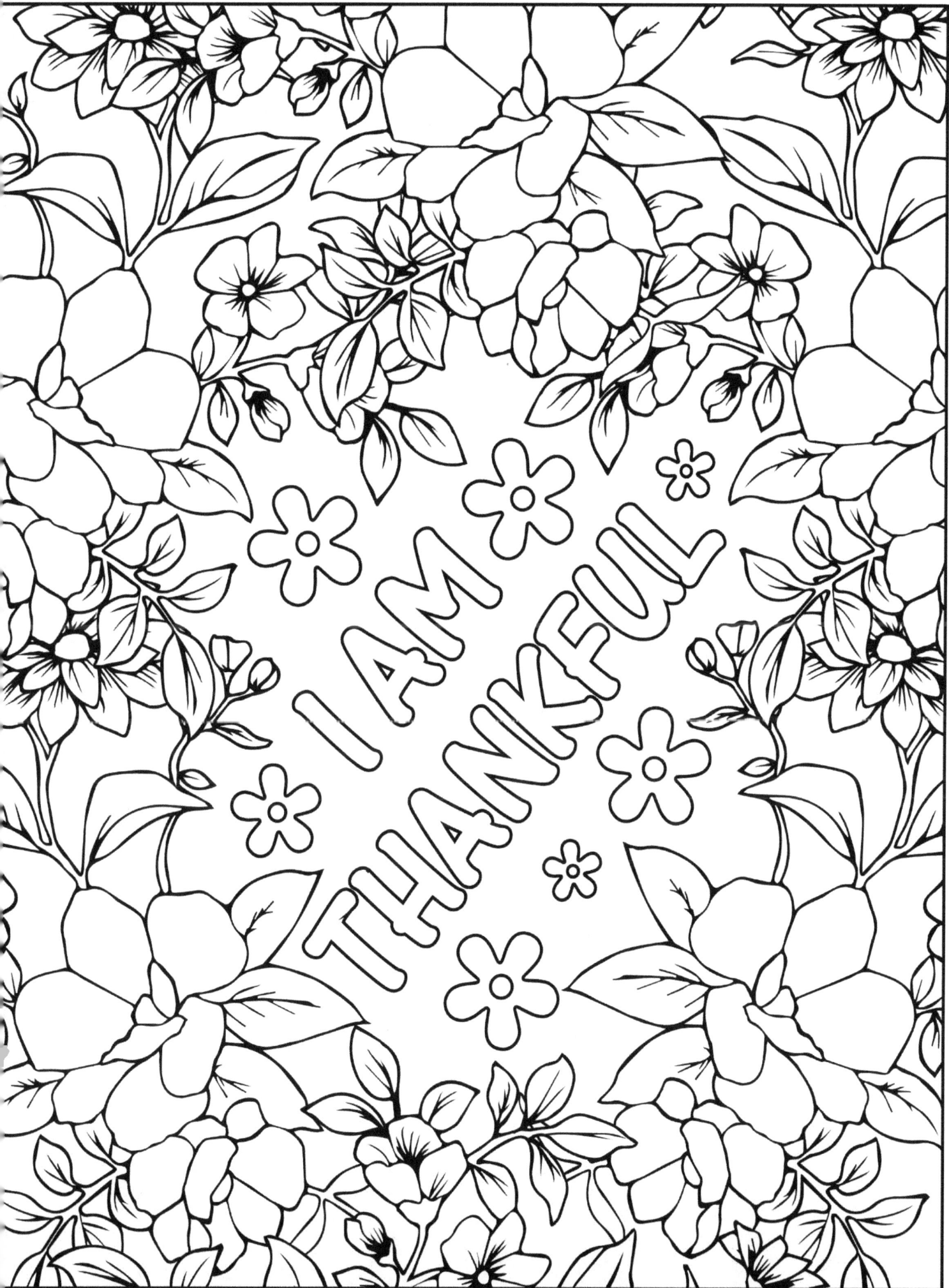

I AM THANKFUL

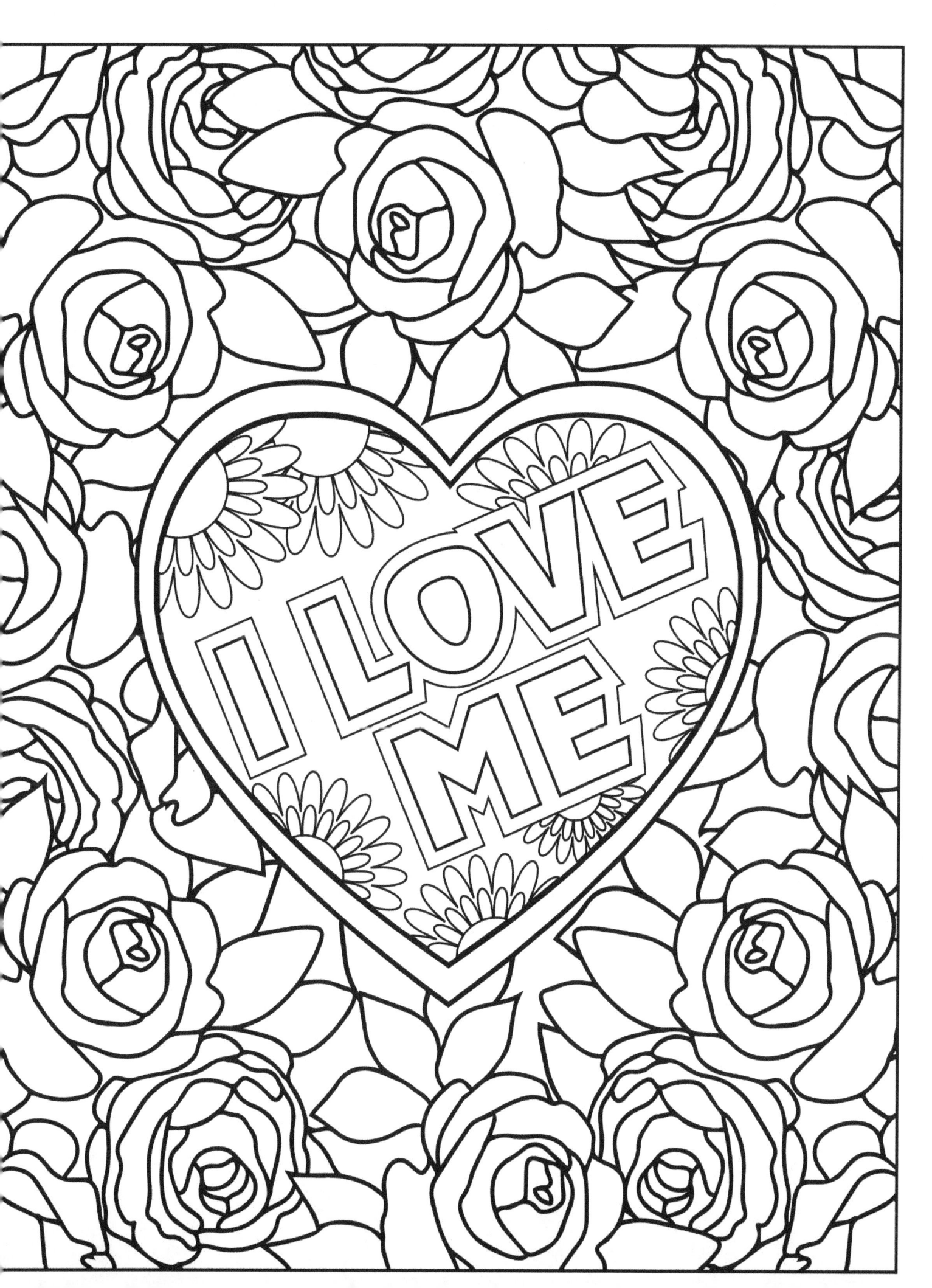

I AM PROUD OF MYSELF

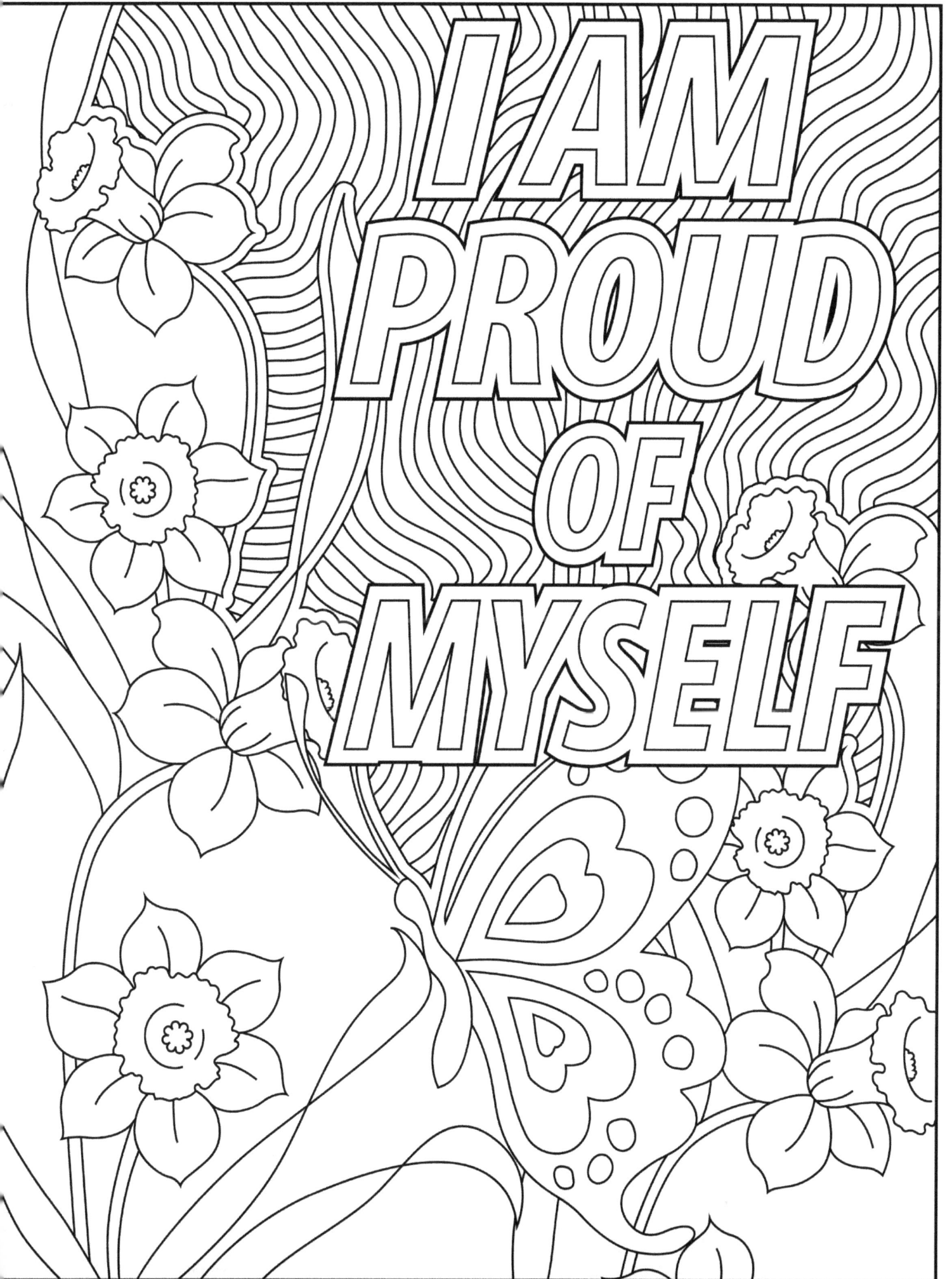

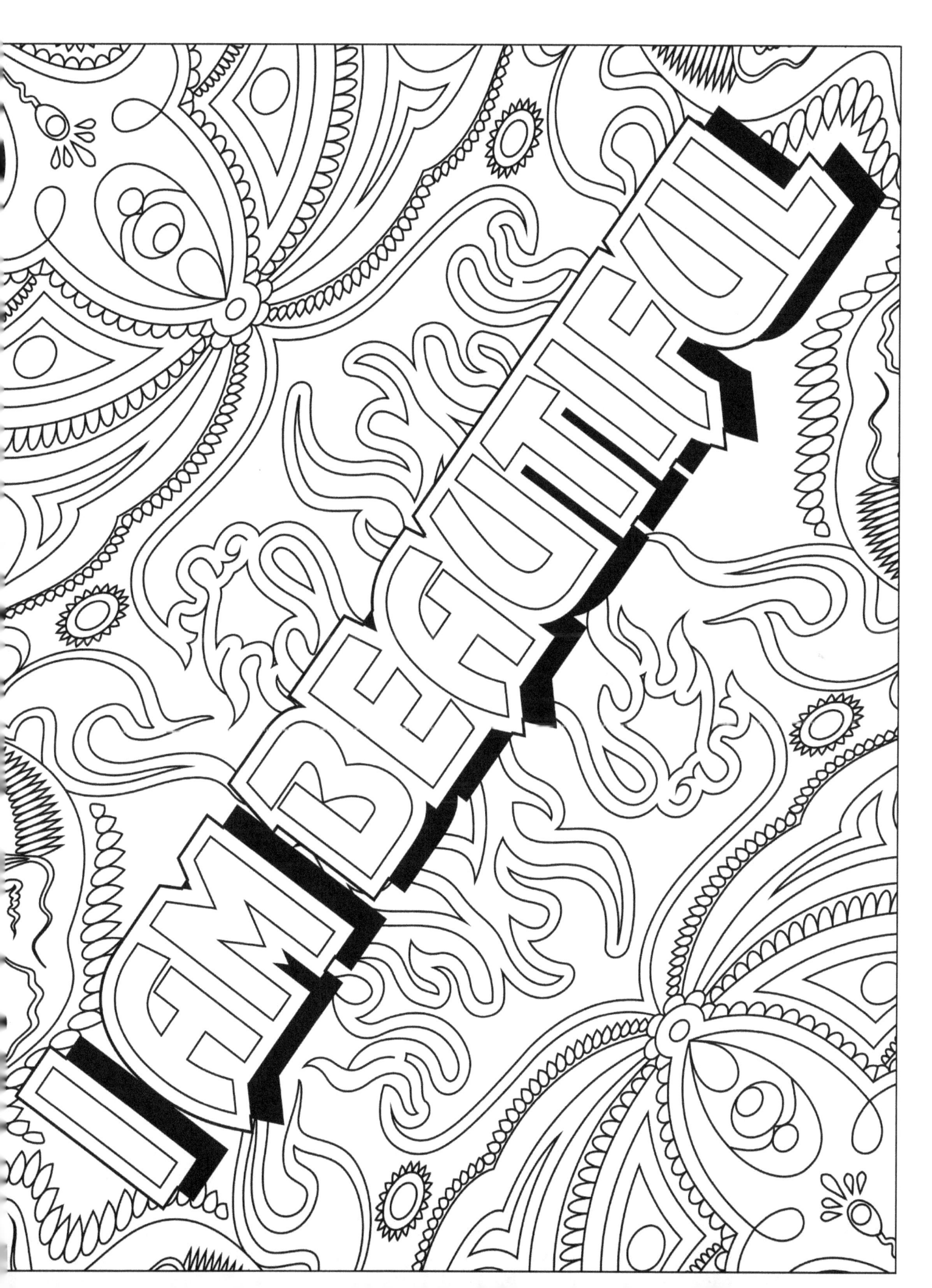

I AM BEAUTIFUL

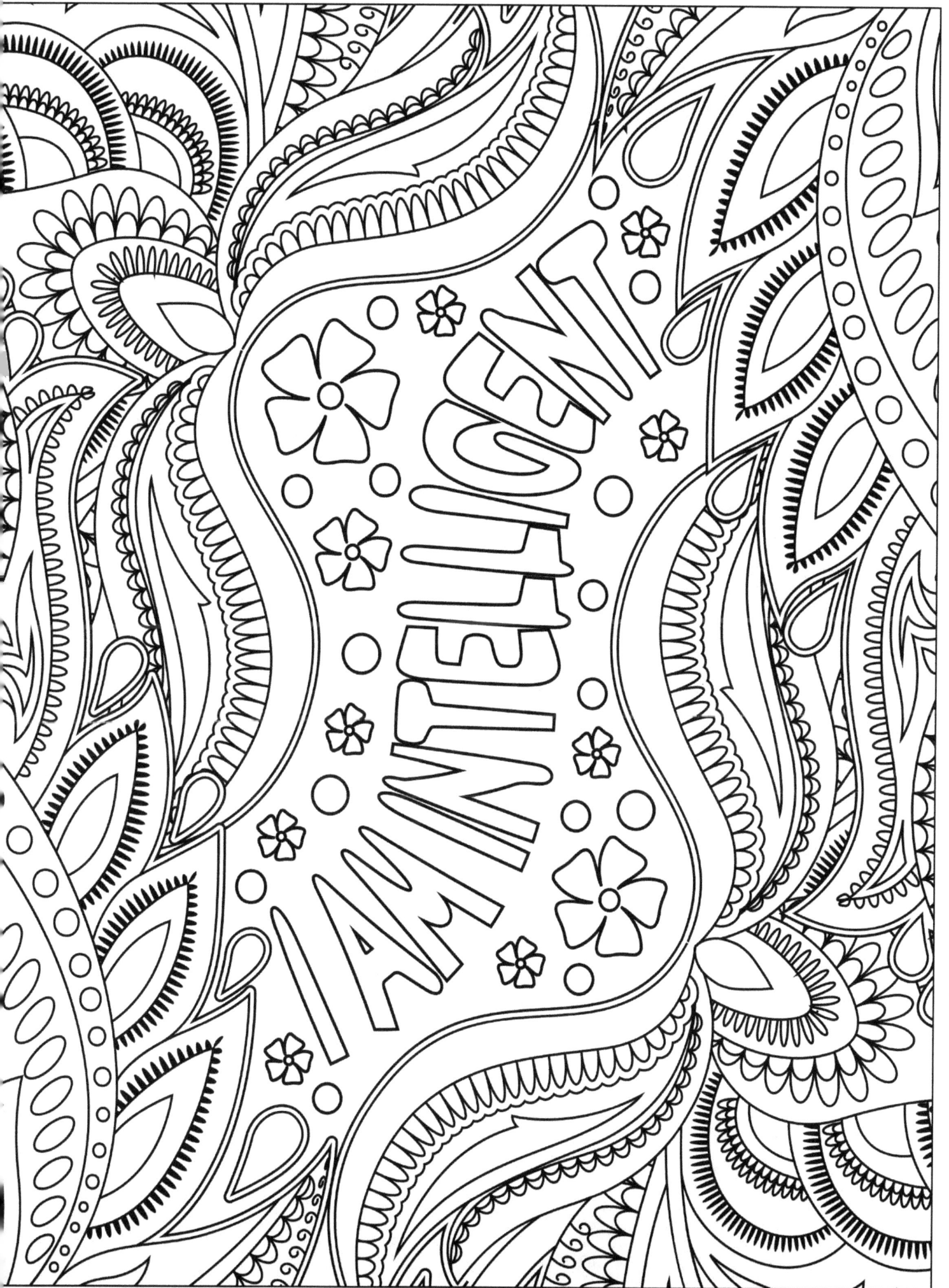

I AM INTELLIGENT

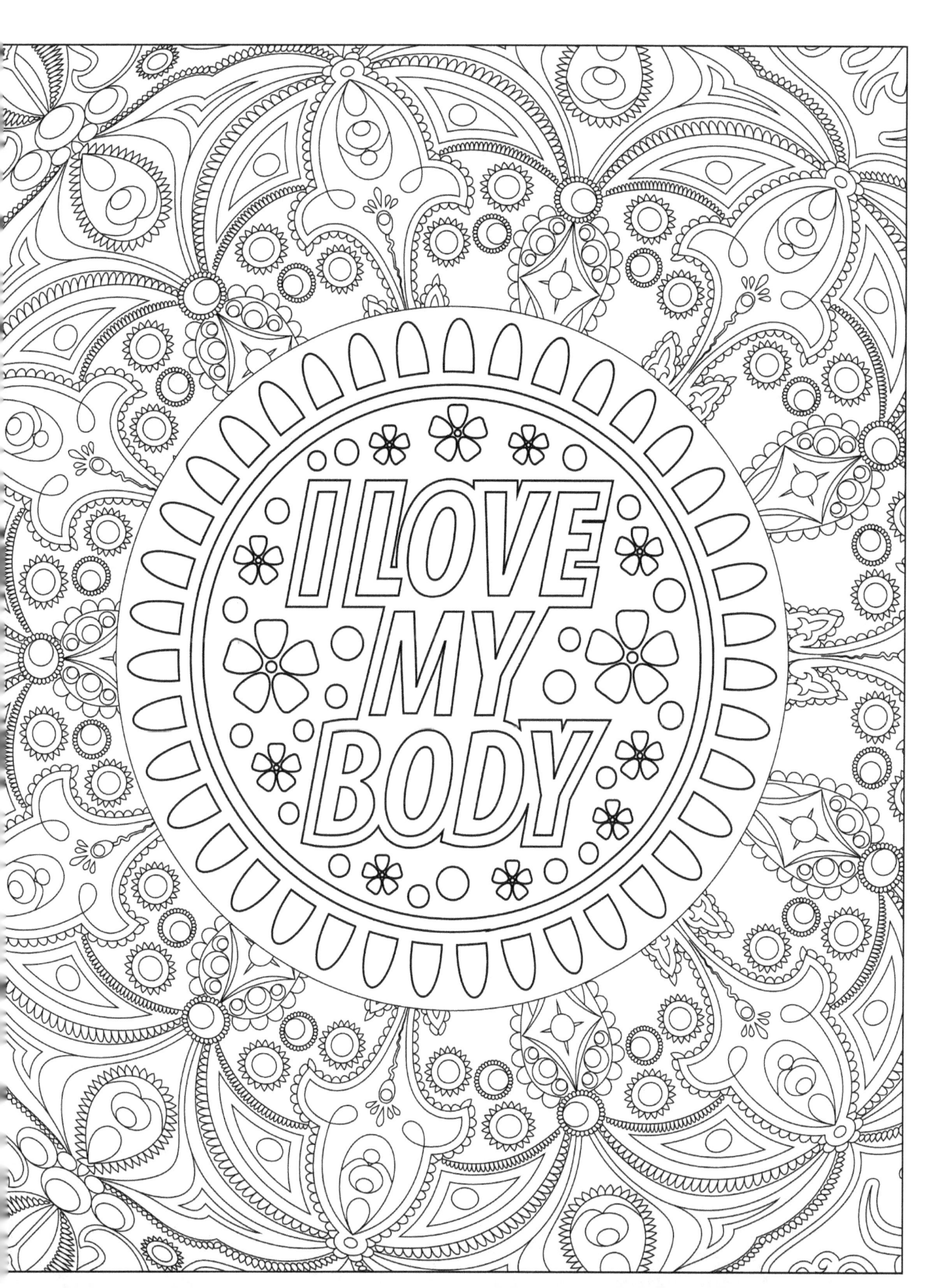

I LOVE MY BODY

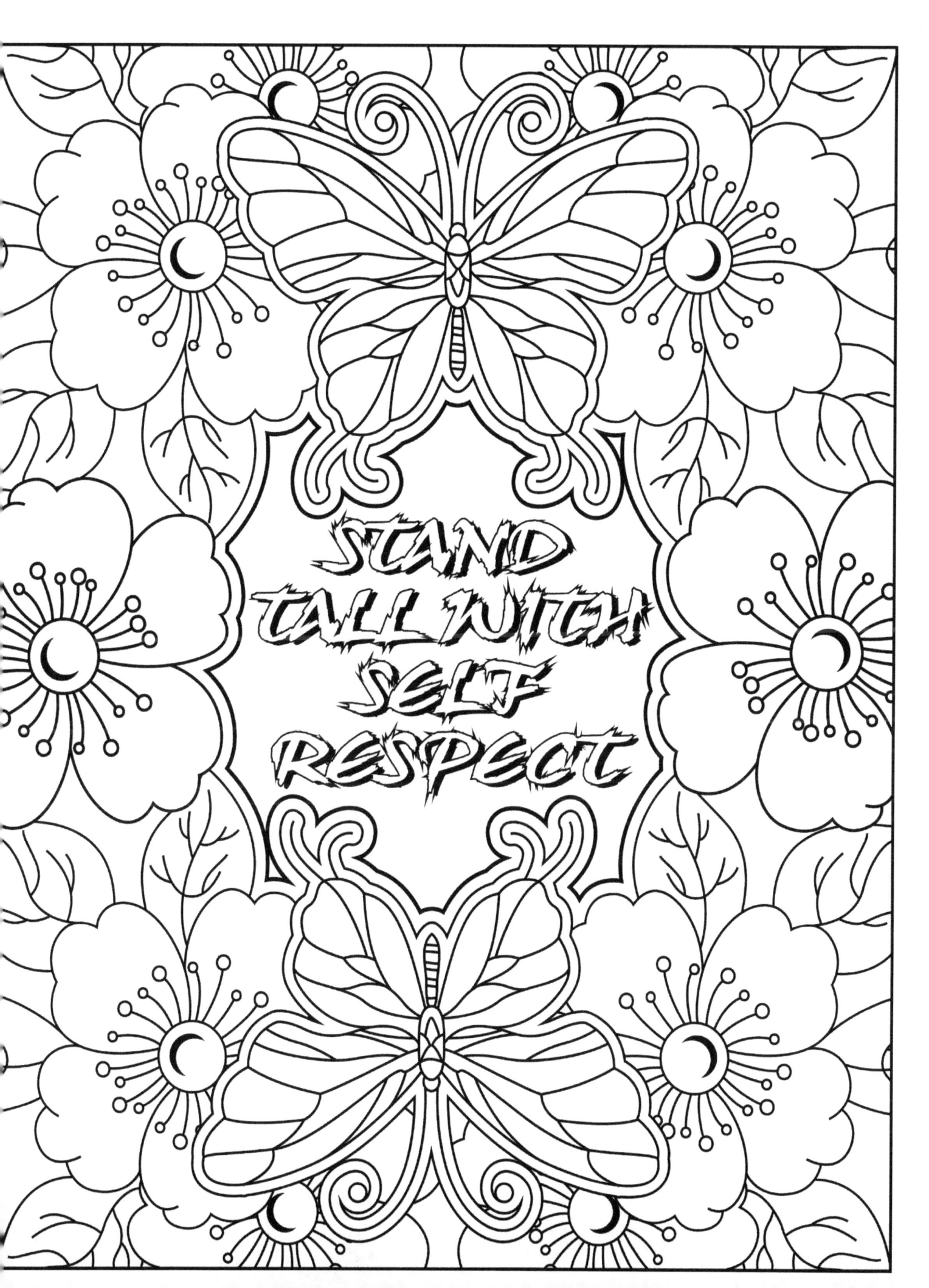

STAND
TALL WITH
SELF
RESPECT

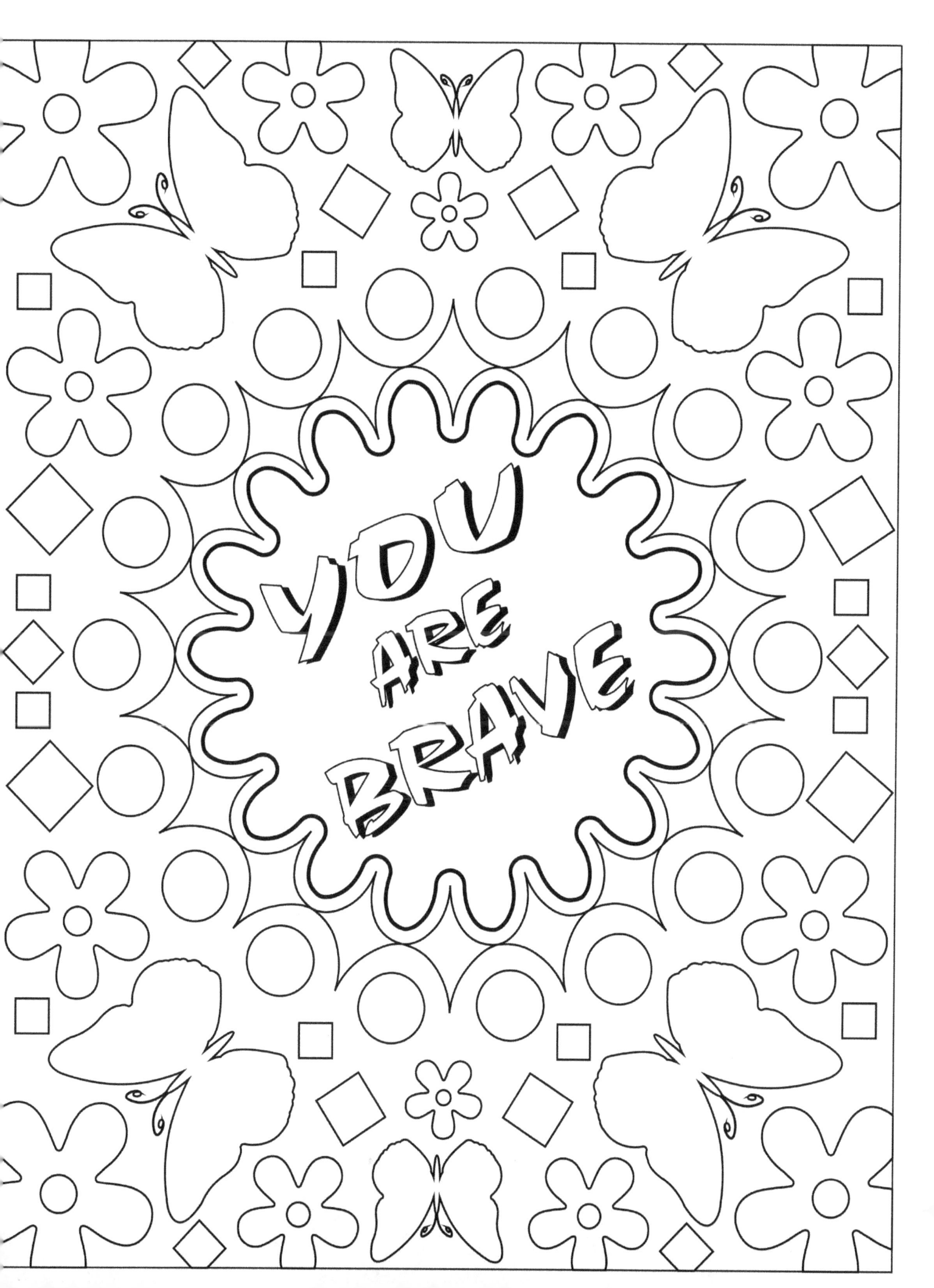

YOU CAN GET THROUGH HARD THINGS

YOU ARE FREE LIKE THE SKY

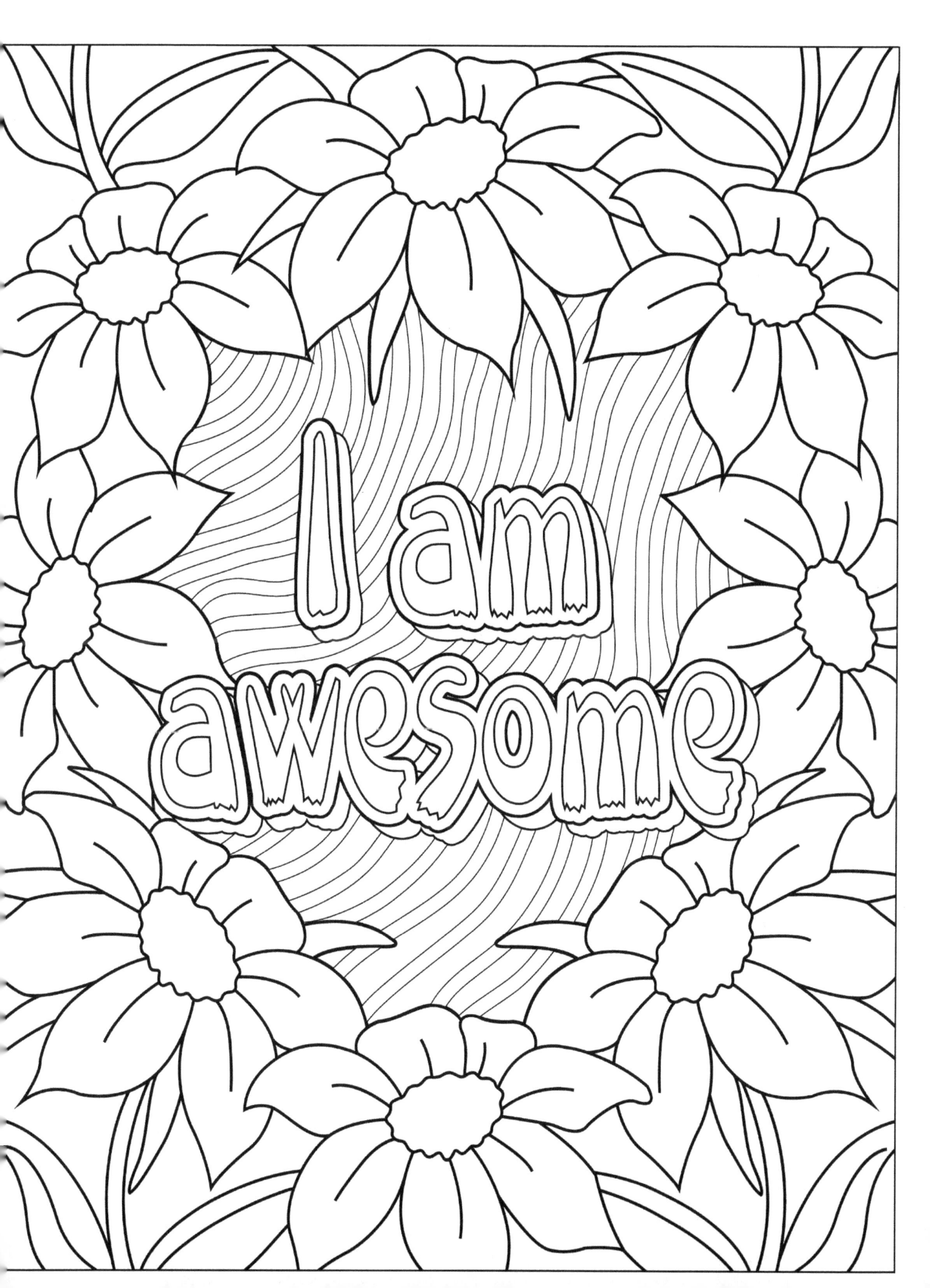

I am awesome

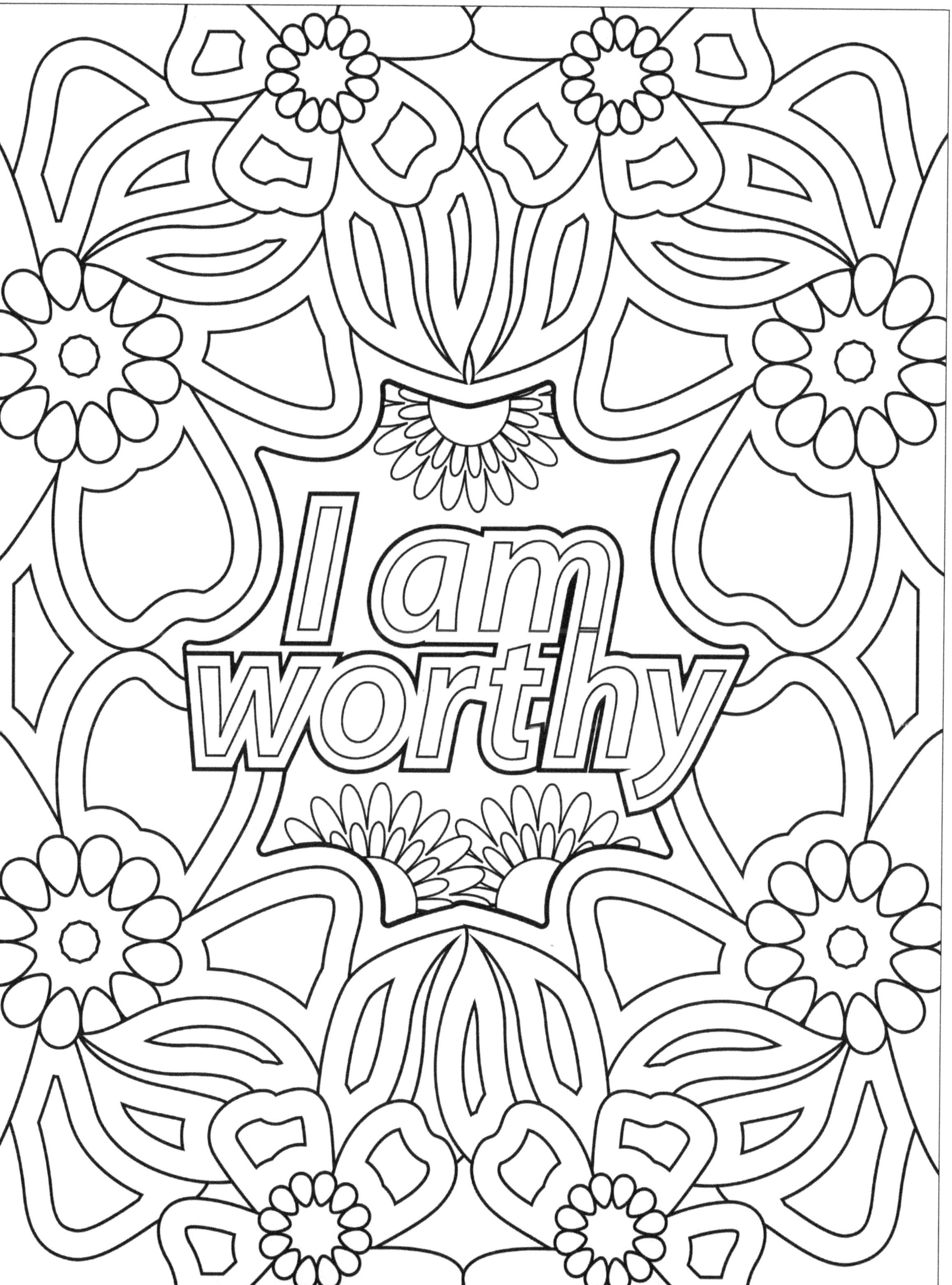

I am worthy

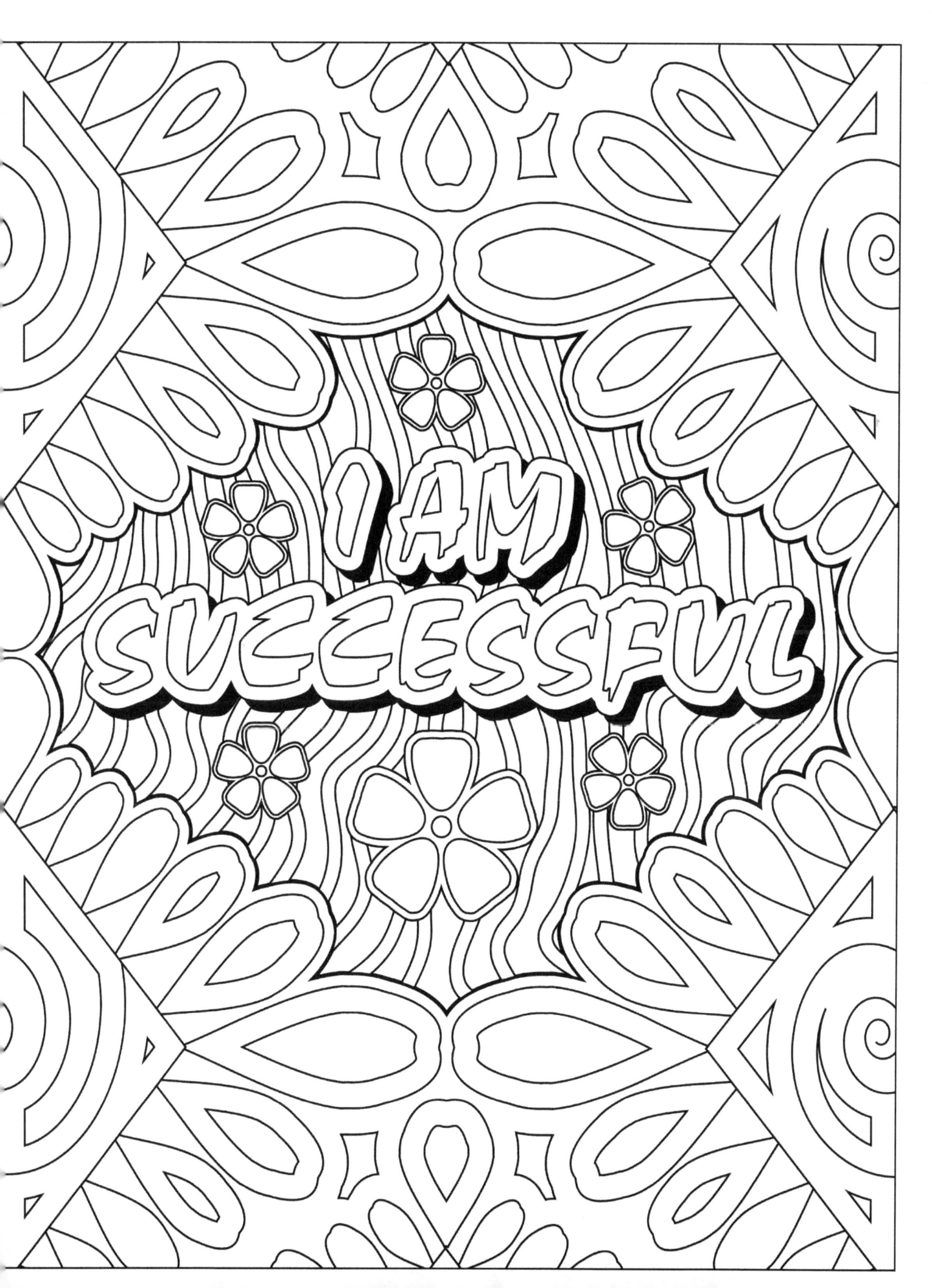

I AM SUCCESSFUL

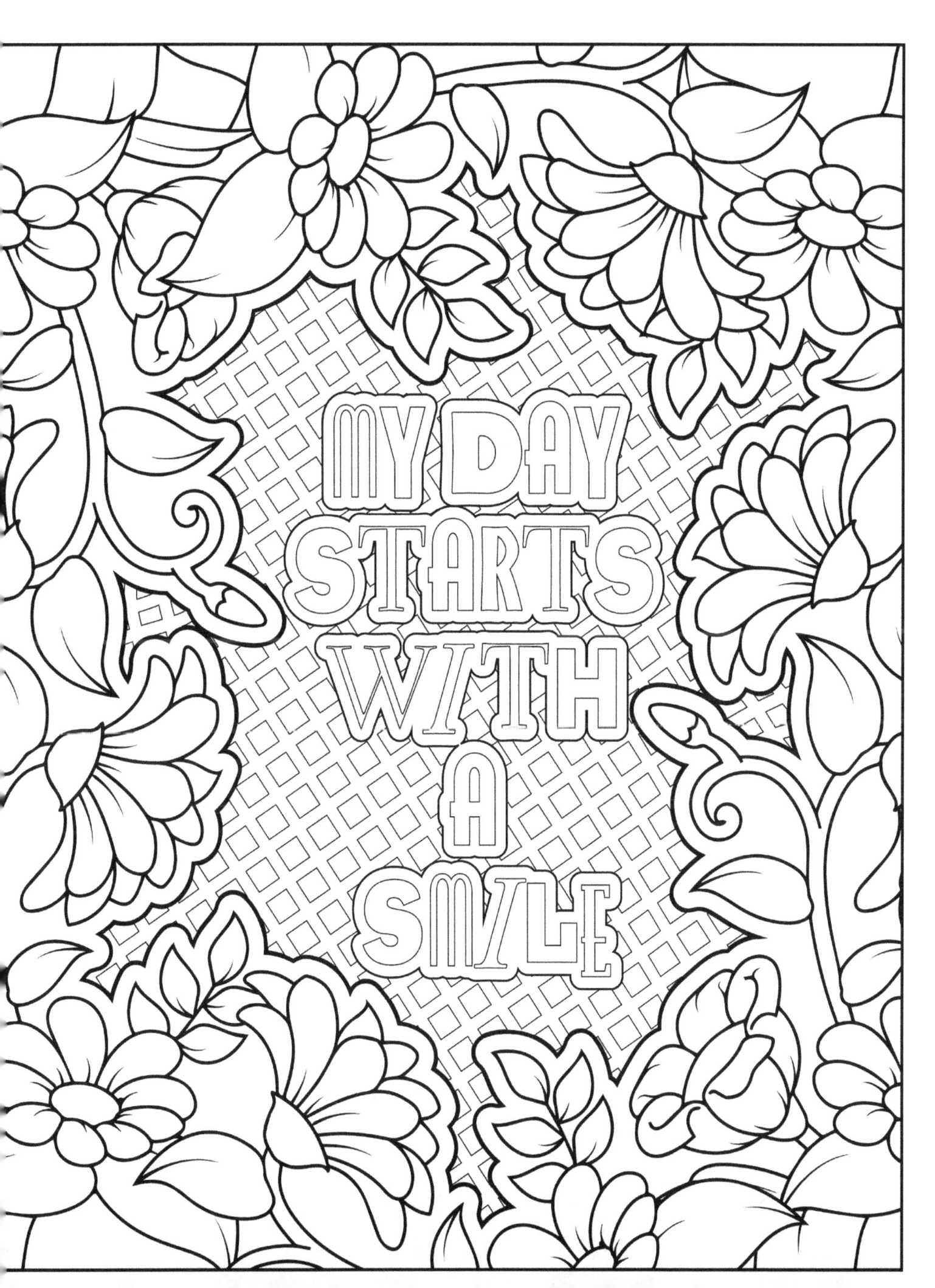

MY DAY STARTS WITH A SMILE

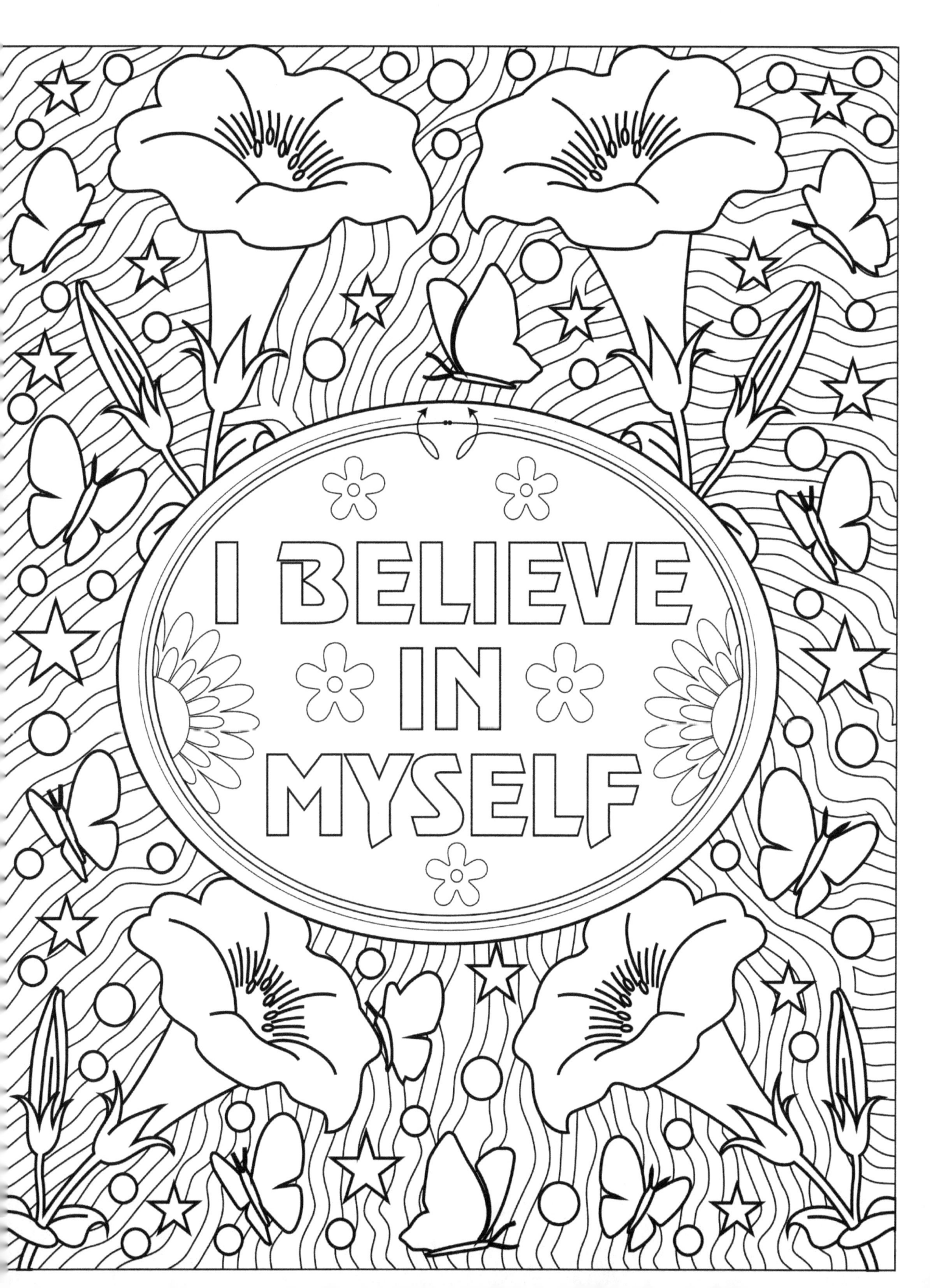

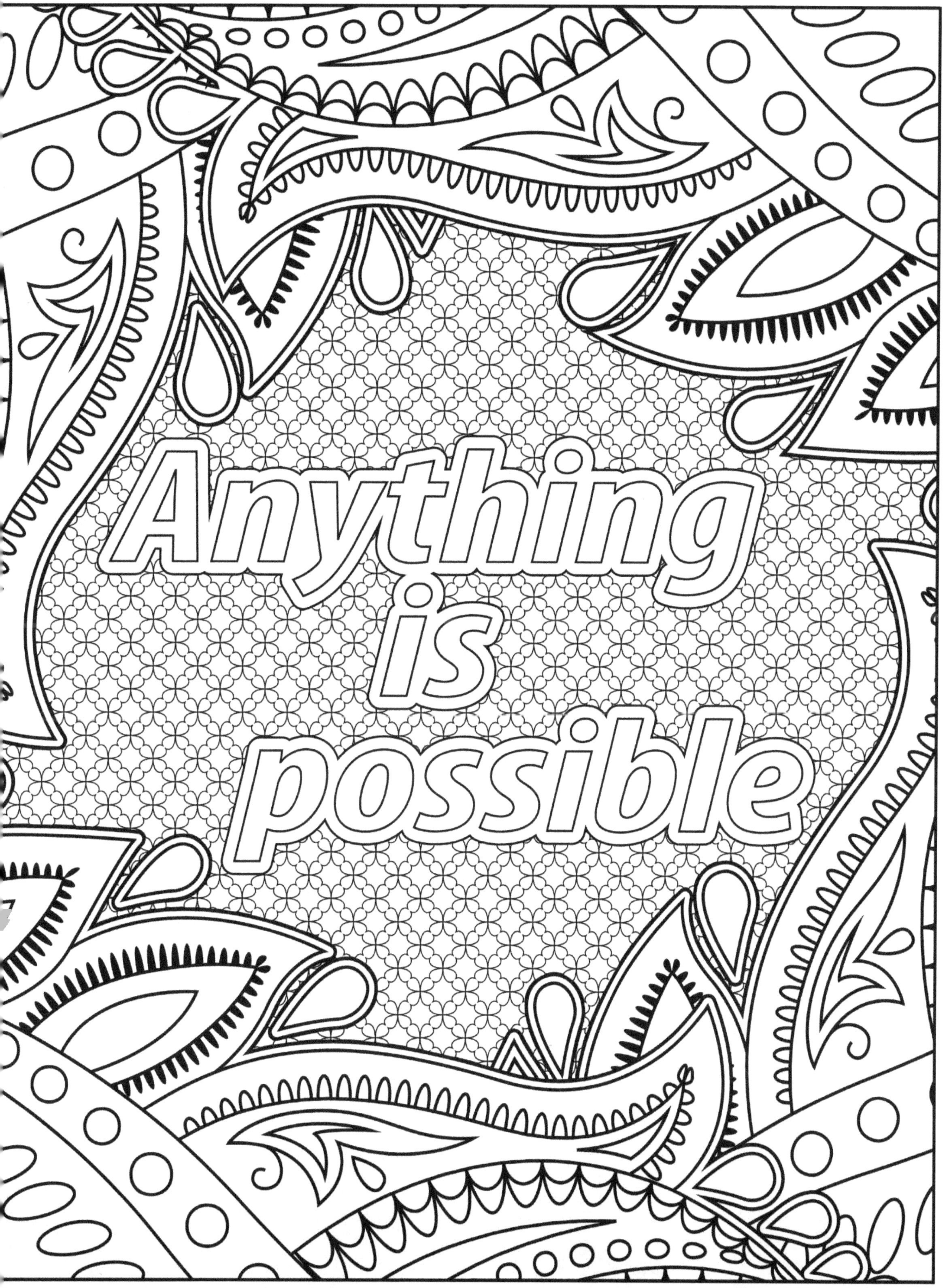

Anything is possible

My
day
starts
with
a
smile

I am happy and healthy

Thank you for purchasing this book.

If you would like to know more about Aryla Publishing Books please visit:-

www.ArylaPublishing.com

Or follow us on
Facebook
Twitter
Instagram
for *free promotions*

@arylapublishing

We would love to know what you think of this book so please leave us a review.

Have a wonderful day ☺

Other Coloring Books from Aryla Publishing

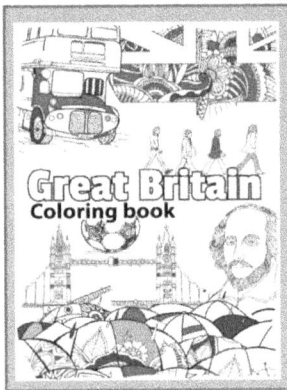

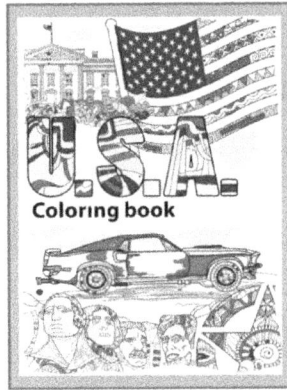

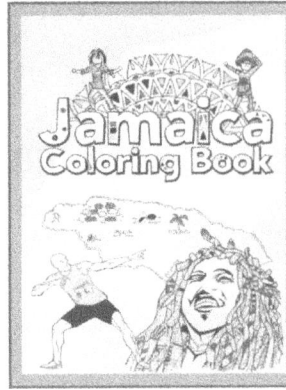

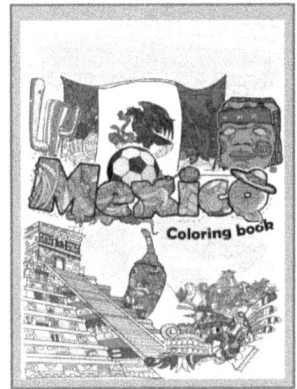

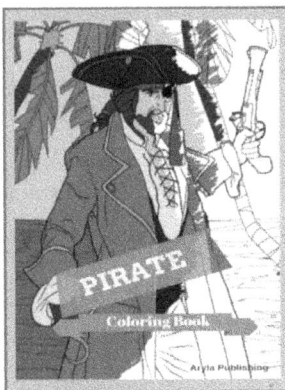

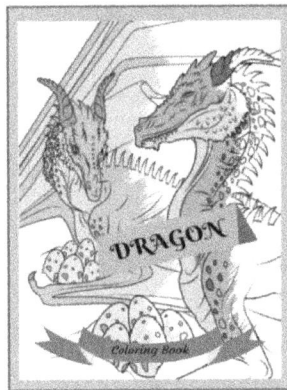

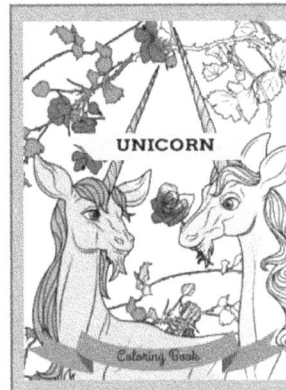

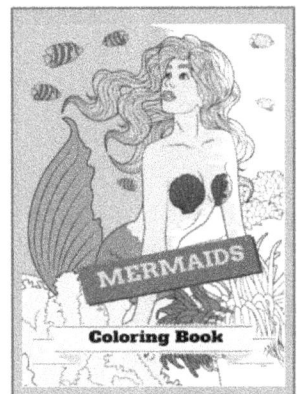

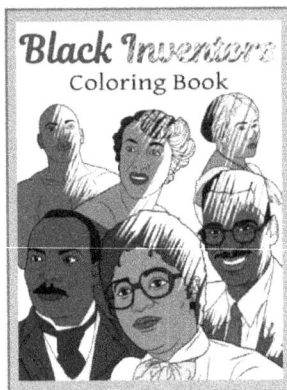

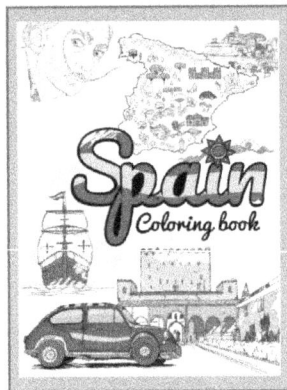

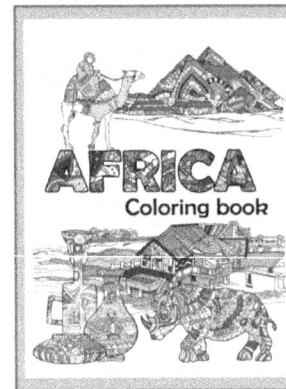

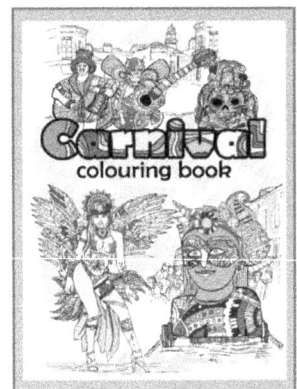

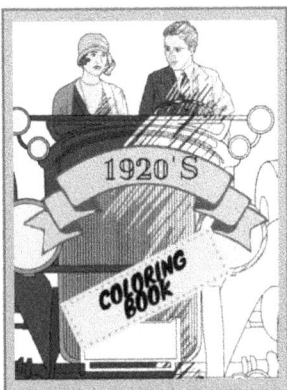

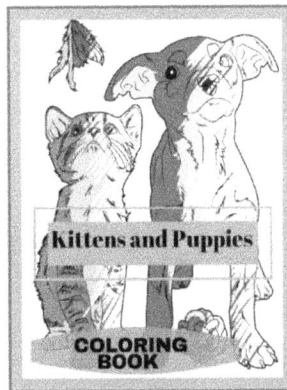

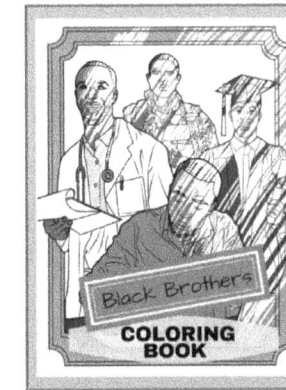

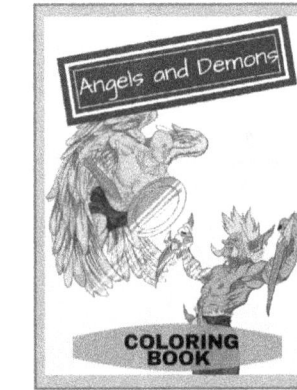

Great Britain Coloring book

U.S.A. Coloring book

Jamaica Coloring Book

Mexico Coloring book

PIRATE Coloring Book

DRAGON Coloring Book

UNICORN Coloring Book

MERMAIDS Coloring Book

Black Inventors Coloring Book

Spain Coloring book

AFRICA Coloring book

Carnival colouring book

1920'S COLORING BOOK

Kittens and Puppies COLORING BOOK

Black Brothers COLORING BOOK

Angels and Demons COLORING BOOK

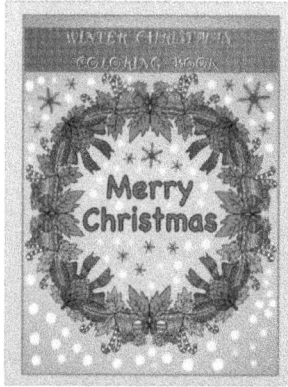
WINTER CHRISTMAS COLORING BOOK
Merry Christmas

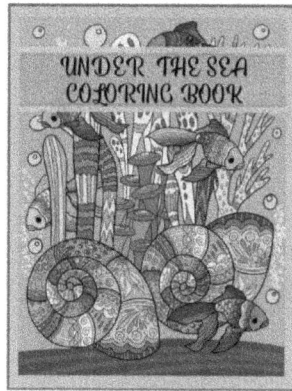
UNDER THE SEA COLORING BOOK

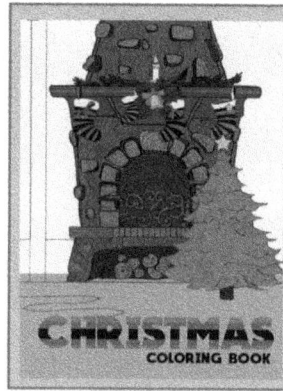
CHRISTMAS
COLORING BOOK

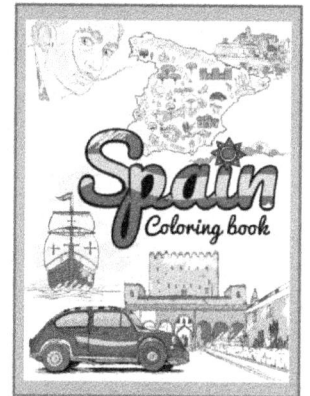
Spain
Coloring book

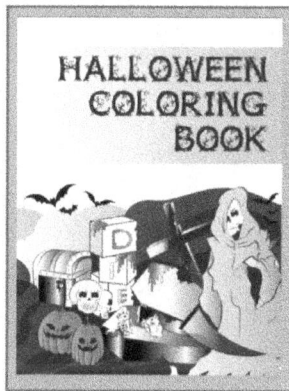
HALLOWEEN COLORING BOOK

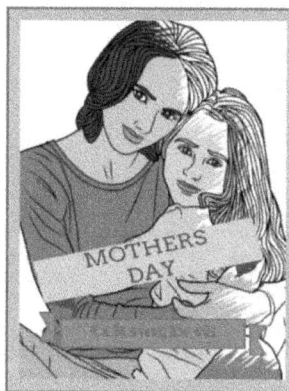
MOTHERS DAY

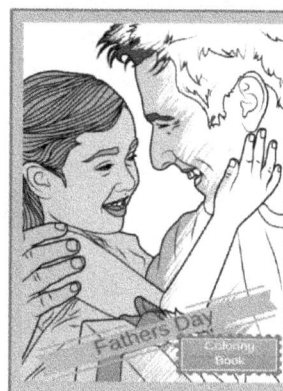
Fathers Day
Coloring Book

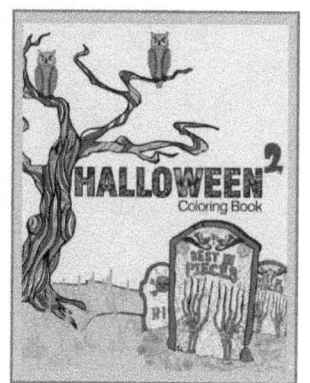
HALLOWEEN²
Coloring Book

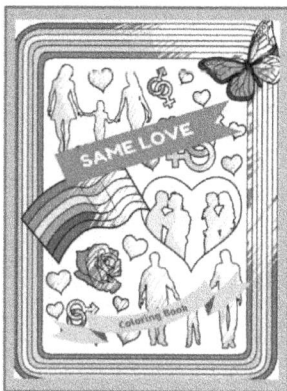
SAME LOVE
Coloring Book

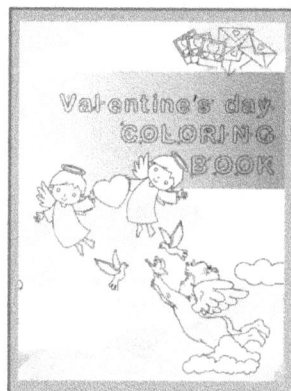
Valentine's day COLORING BOOK

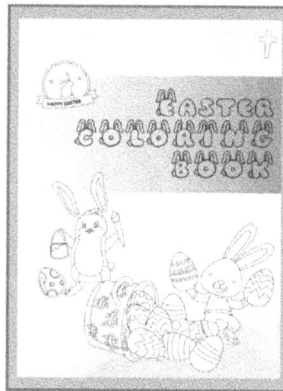
EASTER COLORING BOOK

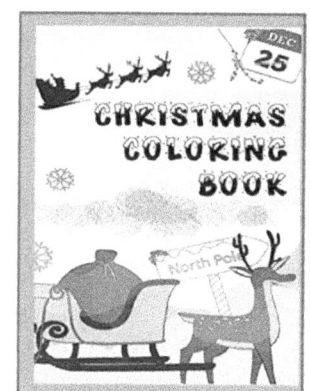
CHRISTMAS COLORING BOOK
North Pole

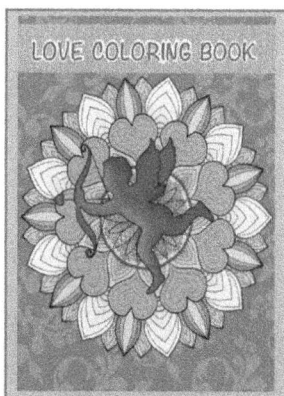
LOVE COLORING BOOK

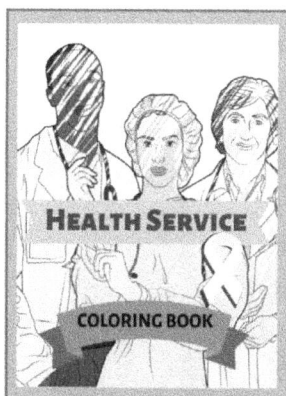
HEALTH SERVICE
COLORING BOOK

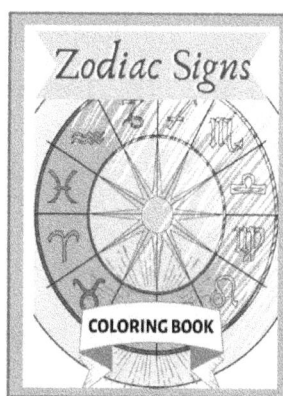
Zodiac Signs
COLORING BOOK

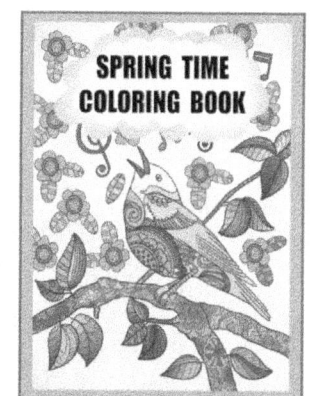
SPRING TIME COLORING BOOK

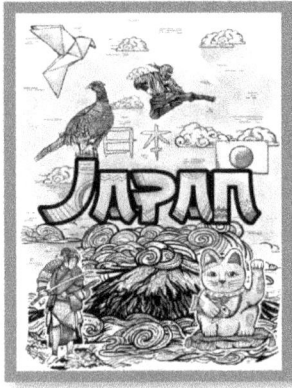

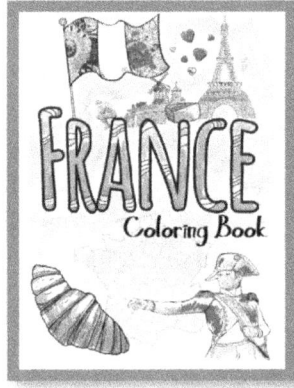

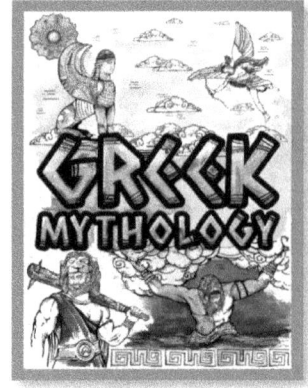

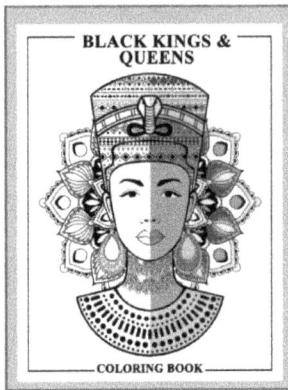

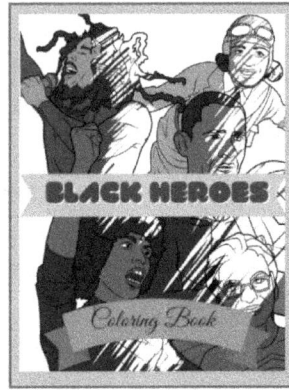

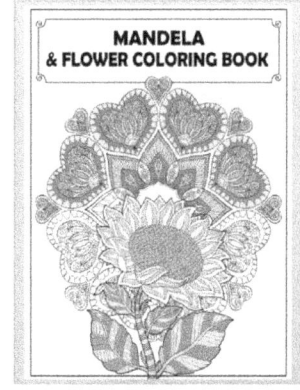

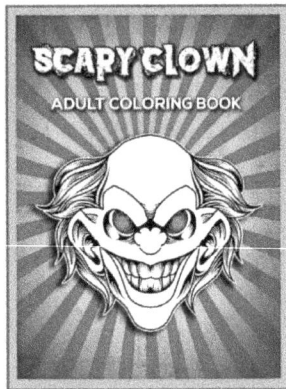

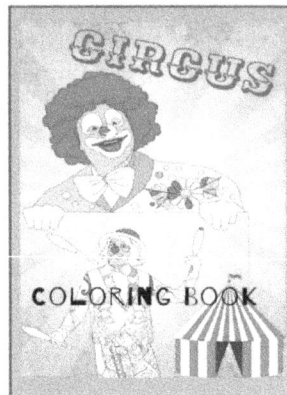

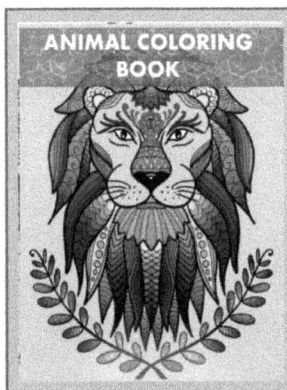

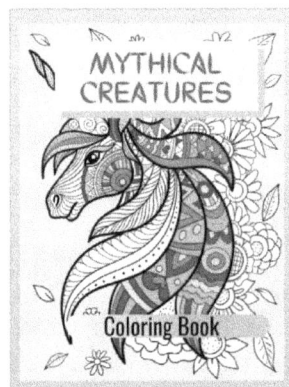

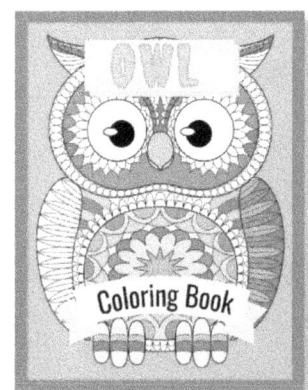

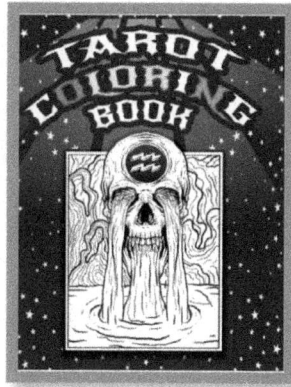
TAROT COLORING BOOK

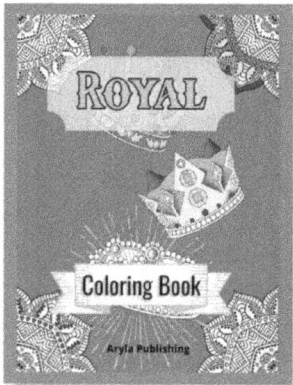
ROYAL Coloring Book
Aryla Publishing

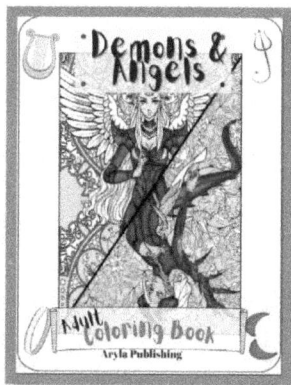
Demons & Angels
Adult Coloring Book
Aryla Publishing

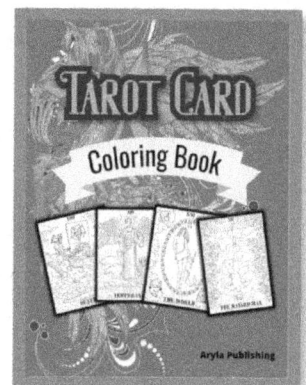
TAROT CARD Coloring Book
Aryla Publishing

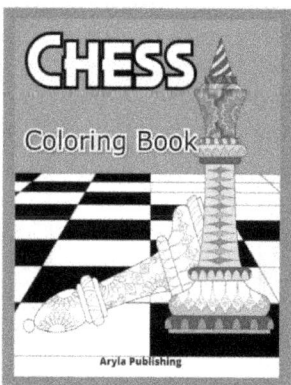
CHESS Coloring Book
Aryla Publishing

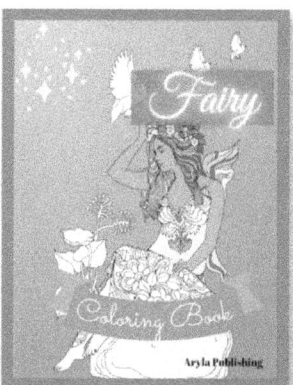
Fairy Coloring Book
Aryla Publishing

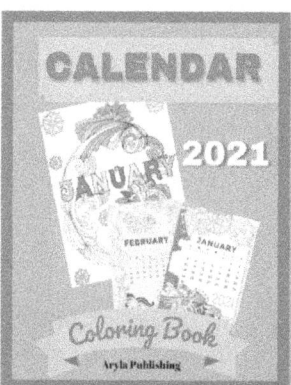
CALENDAR 2021
JANUARY
FEBRUARY   JANUARY
Coloring Book
Aryla Publishing

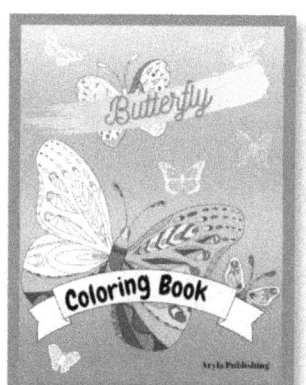
Butterfly Coloring Book
Aryla Publishing

Color In Fun
Kids Books

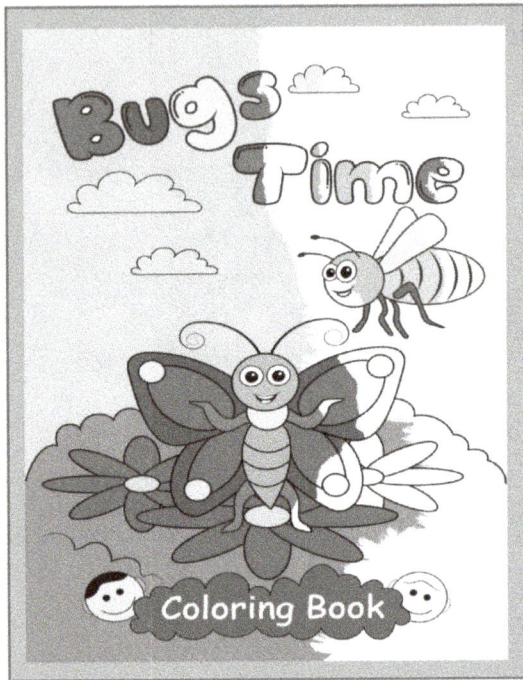

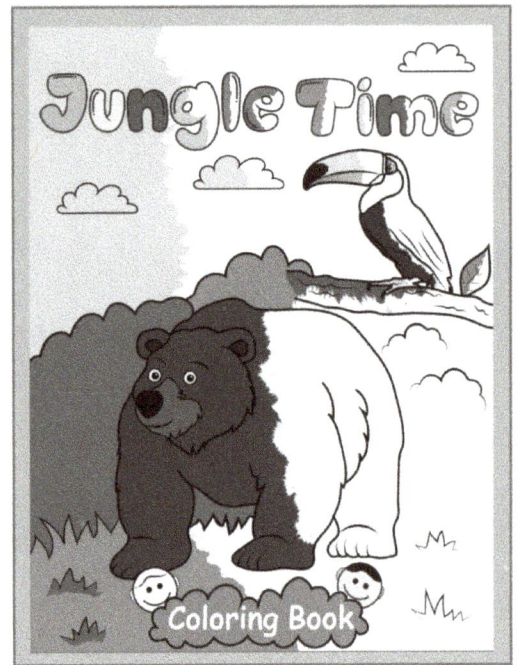

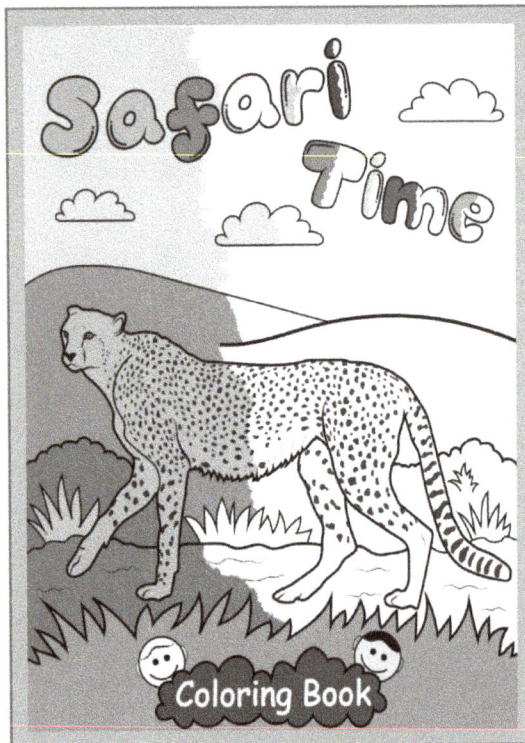

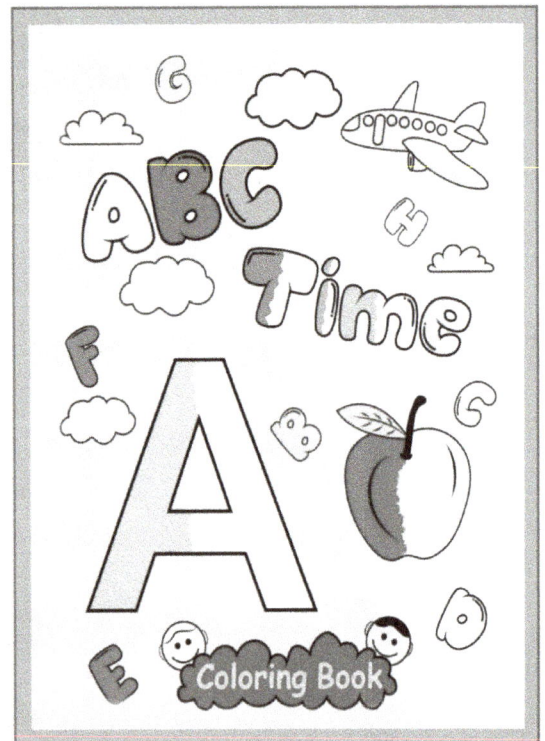

Bugs Time — Coloring Book

Jungle Time — Coloring Book

Safari Time — Coloring Book

ABC Time — Coloring Book

Visit **www.ArylaPublishing.com**
to find out about all new releases.

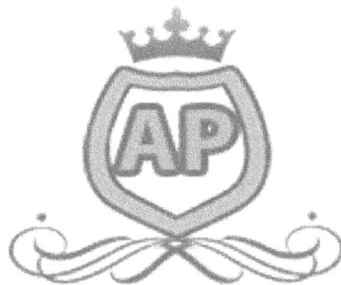

Follow us @arylapublishing on Twitter Instagram & Facebook

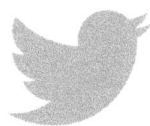

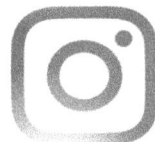

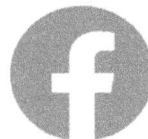

Search for Aryla Publishing on

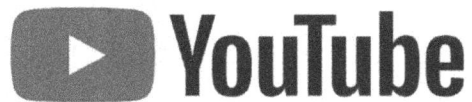

YouTube

Check out our <u>Book Trailers</u>

<u>Subscribe</u> to keep up to date with new releases!

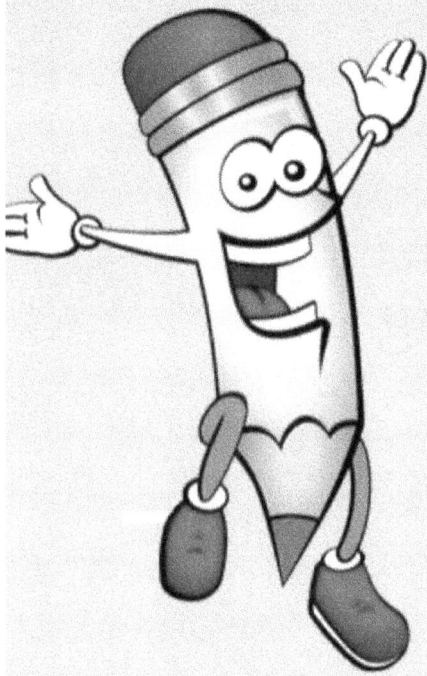

WE WOULD LOVE
YOUR FEEDBACK

PLEASE LEAVE REVIEW AT:-